MENOPAUSE
WHAT EVERY WOMAN NEEDS TO KNOW

YVONNE E. BROOKS

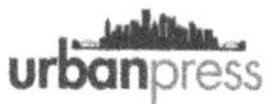

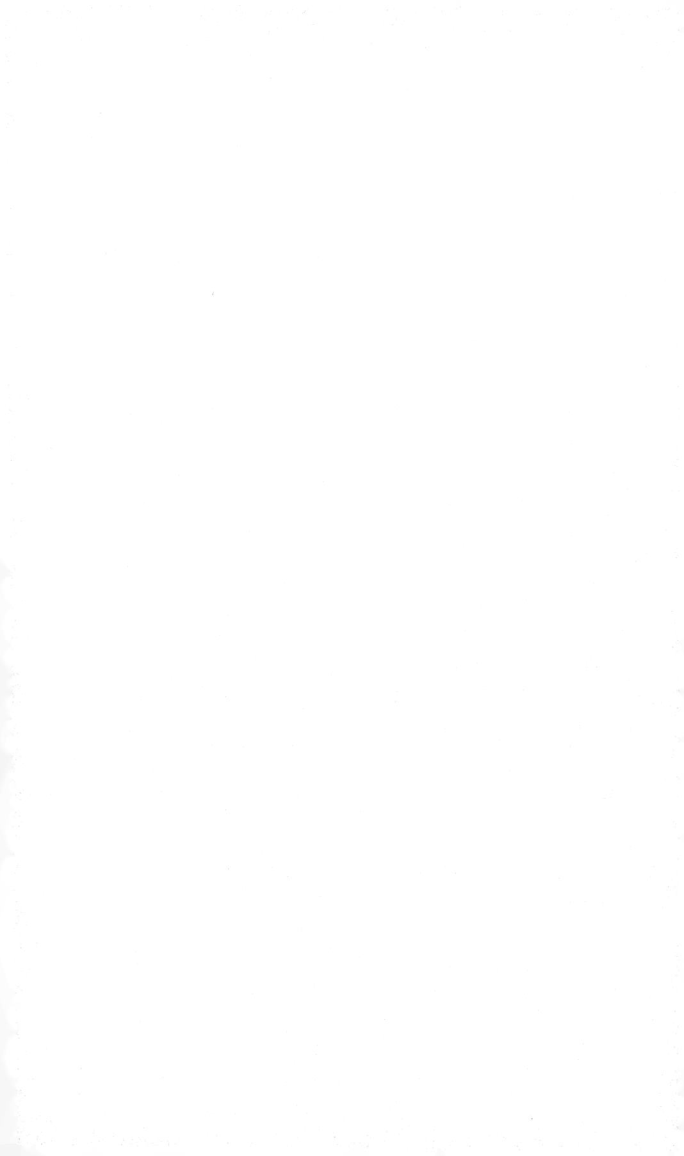

Introduction

Oh menopause, oh menopause,
you're here at last—woohoo!
And all the things I've heard about,
I see you've brought them, too!

Put your feet up, have a brew;
I'm told you're here to stay.
You're going to change my life, I guess;
well, that's what people say.

I've heard that there are lots of things
I'm going to get to meet.
So tell me all about it then;
hang on, I'll take a seat.

Heated flushes, itchy skin,
running to the loo;
Temper tantrums, sleepless nights—
not bad, just to name a few.

Oh, sorry, did you say there's more?
Beg pardon, do go on.
I can't help thinking that's enough;
you surely must be done?

Palpitations, aches and pains,
fluctuating weight;
feeling anxious, stiffening joints—
now let me get this straight.

I have to suffer all of this
because I am a woman?
That's surely just a horrid joke
'cuz most of it's not human!

Night-time sweating, weakened bones;
falling out with friends;
low libido, memory loss—
how long until it ends?

The years may be as long as ten?
Or maybe only five?
But why do I deserve all this?
And how will I survive?

Nagging headaches, always tired,
dryness down below; irritated;
murderous thoughts—
not sure I want to know!

Feeling dizzy, painful boobs,
drying skin and hair;
bloated tummy, thinning nails—
I'm starting to despair!

Don't think I really want to change,
and truly not like this.
It's good you came, but off you go;
I'm giving it a miss.

Muscle tension, burning tongue, low and
tetchy moods. I've heard enough
It sounds like hell
So basically, I'm screwed?!

If women have to cope with this,
then what about the men?
Tell me all the things they will get.
Nothing?!—Say again!

What's that you say, there is one thing;
they do it till their grave.
They have to tend their facial hair;
you mean they have to shave!

Midlife Dramas in Pyjamas
Used with permission.

SYMPTOMS

The last few years have been quite a roller-coaster ride in terms of my personal experience with menopause since I passed through the peri-menopause. If we are married, the reality is that our husbands go on this roller-coaster ride with us without a seat belt. It leaves us (and him) confused, mystified, and frustrated in more ways than one.

I have to confess that this is not a phase in life anyone prepared me for. I didn't even have the awareness to prepare myself. In my mind, it only happened to other people——sorry, other women and I mean old women! Surely, I wasn't old enough for this, and even if I was, how bad could it be? I found out it can be pretty bad.

Whenever I had heard anything about the menopause, it was always treated like a bit of a joke and I assumed the symptoms I heard about would pass me by. I have found in general that most women bury their heads in the sand where menopause is concerned, believing it won't happen to them or they will get lucky and miss it altogether. Such is not the case.

Recently, I was invited to give a talk on the subject. The organiser told me afterwards that she struggled to get women to attend since most didn't see what it had to do with them. They also found the topic embarrassing. Even the lady asked to introduce it did not want to do it, so the group leader had to introduce me. Maybe we think if we avoid the subject, we will not to experience it or it will just go away. I assure you, it will not.

This roller-coaster ride has not been the easiest thing I have ever done, but I found that gathering information and talking about it openly and privately with women and men have smoothed my passage and put me in a position to help other women, even if only a little. There are things we can do to prepare for this season of life and I want to share those with you, along with my experience as well as the experiences of some of my friends and associates willing to share their stories.

Without exception, every woman I have spoken to about this subject has said they thought they were the only one going through it. That is the reason I asked other women to join me in sharing a little of their story, too. I asked many to share, but only a few responded, even though they all had a story. I am grateful to those who contributed, and you will read their stories in the last chapter.

In the Introduction, you read a light-hearted poem about this serious subject and it included many symptoms that usually surprise the inexperienced on uninformed, for most believe hot flashes and a cessation of the menstrual cycle are the main characteristics of menopause. Here are some of the other symptoms I experienced, and many were unnerving and surprising:

- Hot feet;
- Various types of flushes/flashes;
- Profuse sweating (from everywhere);
- Interrupted sleep;
- Frequent urination/irritable bladder;
- Extremely itchy and dry skin;
- Weak, fragile nails on hands; thickening nails on feet;
- Hair growth on chin (may as well say I grew a beard);
- Breaking, thinning dry hair on head;
- Olefactory changes relating to the sense of smell;
- Changes in the palate and my sense of taste;
- Visual and auditory changes (although I cannot say if these particular changes are due to age or the menopause).

Let me be more specific about some of these symptoms of "the change of life" as some have called it.

I experienced hot flushes (implosions and explosions) that also included burning hot feet like I was walking on hot coals or like someone had rubbed chili peppers on my skin—and that included my face, neck, chest, arms, and legs. At other times, I had a sensation like someone had thrown petrol over me and then lit it with a torch.

My sleep was interrupted by frequent visits to the toilet, especially during the night. At other times, my thinking was foggy, and my memory became so erratic that I started thinking I was experiencing dementia. Once when speaking in a public forum, I had the strangest sensation of having my thoughts highlighted and cut out without them being pasted anywhere else in my memory. This left me not remembering what I had just said or what I wanted to say next. For the first time in my life, I felt panic when I spoke and, as a result, I didn't accept speaking engagements for a few months.

What's more, I did not enjoy taking a

shower in public while I was fully dressed, which was what it felt like as the perspiration poured from my face, running down my chin, arms, and legs. I realised after a short while that if I gave in to the panic, I would lose my nerve and maybe lay the groundwork for more serious mental health problems regarding panic/anxiety attacks

I began writing everything down, making copious lists——that is, if I could still remember what I wanted to write down by the time I found a pen and paper. I experienced sweating from parts of my body I didn't even know had sweat glands, even in my head. This of course impacted the condition of my hair, which was dripping wet most of the time and caused me concern for my hair breaking or falling out.

I have been blessed with one of the most talented and skilled hairdressers in the world. She has been tremendous, caring for my hair and making sure I had treatments like dying my grey roots and then not dying my grey roots when I decided to let the natural highlights grow through. I didn't make a conscious decision about my eyebrows, however, and wasn't really aware they were growing grey until I went to have them threaded. I instructed the beautician to pick out the few greys that were there. She informed me that if she did that, I would have no eyebrows. I informed her that I didn't need to pay to get insulted as I could get that service at home for free.

Whilst I was concerned about losing the hair on my head, I had no such worries about the hair on my chin. What had started off when I was twenty as one hair on the left side of my chin grew into a full beard. Fortunately but painfully, I started threading my chin, which expanded to include my neck and upper lip. I made the decision ahead of time that once I can no longer take the pain, I will definitely become the bearded lady and join the next circus that comes to town. My hairdresser encouraged me to keep going and helped me hold on to my sanity.

Oh yes, and the other thing is that I actually felt like I was going out of your mind, coupled with a sense of fatigue and exhaustion that was at times overwhelming.

I am not writing this as any kind of authority on this subject apart from my own personal journey. I want to share my experience with others who are interested and may benefit from what I went through. Every woman I have spoken to has expressed the thought that while she was going into this season, she felt she was the only one who felt this way. I want you, my dear reader, to know that you are not alone——and if you are a man, to know what your partner or loved one is going through. Let's get started in the next chapter talking a bit about what exactly the menopause is.

2

What is the Menopause?

Maybe the question should be what is peri-menopause because actual menopause is a little further down the road. Peri-menopause is a normal part of life, just like puberty (the onset of your first period). Menopause is the time of your last period, but symptoms usually begin several years before that, thus the term peri-menopause. What's more, these symptoms can last for months or even years after your final period. They commence around 40 years of age but can begin any time after 35 (or sooner if you have your womb and ovaries removed through a hysterectomy and oophorectomy).

At first, you may notice that your monthly periods become more erratic or occur more (or less) often. They may last longer, become heavier, and vary in frequency. Sometimes without warning, you find yourself feeling very warm at any time during the day or night. It could feel like someone has turned up the heat after closing all the windows. You will know you have entered peri-menopause when one of the songs you sing the most has the words "is it hot in here or is it just me?" in every line. This is caused by the fluctuations in the levels of oestrogen and progesterone, the two female hormones produced in your ovaries.

Peri means that you are "in the area of" menopause, usually beginning several years before your last menstrual period. It lasts for approximately one year after your last period, and this is the point known as menopause. At least one full year without a period is needed before you can say you have been "through menopause." Post menopause follows peri-menopause when you are no longer fertile, which lasts for the rest of your life. For many women, this is great news since it means they no longer have to worry about getting pregnant or having periods. At the same time, for many of those women, they can no longer remember what they did to get pregnant.

Menopause doesn't usually occur before a woman is forty, but it can happen any time from our thirties to our mid-fifties or later. The average age for it to occur is when we are fifty-one—but don't be surprised if it shows up when it is good and ready to do so, and not according to anyone's prediction or schedule.

If you were or are a smoker, you can experience early menopause. It can also be brought on by a surgery, like the removal (hysterectomy) of the womb, also known as the uterus or the baby factory. This will end your periods, but if your ovaries are not removed, you will carry on producing hormones. That means you could still have symptoms of menopause when your ovaries start to produce less oestrogen. If, however, both ovaries are removed (oophorectomy), menopausal symptoms can be immediate regardless of your age since you have lost your main supplier of oestrogen.

What Are the Signs of Menopause?

Since no two women are the same, the signs and symptoms vary from woman to woman because oestrogen is used by many parts of our bodies. Therefore, changes in how much oestrogen we have available can cause a variety of symptoms. There are so many symptoms that it's not possible for any one woman to have them all or even the majority of them——at least that's my prayer for you.

Everything you experience as you go through menopause may be a byproduct of getting older. (Yes, I know that has really made your day, but look on the bright side: Getting older is better than the alternative of *not* getting older.)

Changes in your period might be the symptom you notice first. Your period may become irregular. How much blood you lose could also change and it may become lighter or heavier than normal. Your periods may also be shorter or longer, due to normal changes in your reproductive system as you go through the change. You should see your doctor if:

- your periods come very close together;
- you have heavy bleeding;
- you have spotting between periods;
- your periods last more than a week.

Hot flushes are quite common and are one of the more obvious symptoms of menopause, and they are due to the changes in our hormones. Unfortunately, the hot flashes can last a few years after menopause. I was under the impression they would immediately disappear, but speaking to older women and from my own experience, they can hang around long after the party is over. I have noticed, however, that those later flushes are not as severe and that the sweating is minimal.

The dictionary says "a hot flash is a sudden, intense feeling of heat in the top half or even all of one's body." The first heat symptoms I experienced were in my feet. The heat was so intense that I actually checked my feet for blisters since it felt like I had been walking on hot coals. I had to resort to sleeping with my feet out from under the sheets at night. It's funny that I never felt that symptom during the daytime. After a few months of that, I started to get the full-body flushes. I then started my quest to find someone who could tell me precisely when this would end. I am still looking.

Your face and neck can feel as though they have become a radiator so that others can literally warm their hands from the heat you produce——at least they could with me. My glasses would actually fog up in cold weather. Your face can become flushed and blotches may appear on your chest, back, and arms. Heavy sweating can ensue.

Later in my journey, I experienced

freezing cold flushes that were so bad, they left me longing for a hot flush, but just like the buses, one never came when I needed it. Flushes can be mild, feeling like a warm, Caribbean sea breeze, or severe enough to wake you from a deep sleep (this is referred to as night sweats). In my case, it sometimes felt I had been plunged into a vat of boiling oil. The hot flushes would last between 30 seconds and 10 minutes—and I know because I timed them. It was like riding a wave, which went from my feet upwards to my head. It was like I had fallen off my surfboard and plunged into the ocean.

Many nights I would be boiling hot and throw the covers off, only to wake up later freezing cold and trying to steal heat from my husband's body. By then, I am sure he thought I had lost my mind. I would wake up and throw the windows wide open in the middle of winter, only to wake up later shivering and wondering which mad person had opened the windows in the middle of winter.

There was no happy medium because once I started to warm up, my internal thermostat would blow up and I would end up overheating again. Many mornings I woke up feeling exhausted like I had been working in the mines with the seven dwarfs "all night long"——a la Lionel Ritchie.

As if I have not discouraged you enough already, there are more symptoms I learned about as I talked to other women, some of which I experienced firsthand, some not. I suspect the same will be true for you, so I include them in the next chapter just so you are aware of them, while hoping you never experience them.

Problems With Your Vagina and Bladder

Changing oestrogen levels can cause your genital area to get drier and the skin thinner, which could cause you to experience extreme itching, which can then lead to endless scratching and irritation. Dryness of the vagina can make sexual intercourse very uncomfortable. You can get around this, however, by using a lubricant recommended by your pharmacist or prescribed by your GP.

You may think you have a thrush infection, but this is rare unless you suffer from diabetes or you are on a high dose of antibiotics, which could trigger it. You can speak to your GP who may be willing to prescribe a hormonal cream that will relieve the irritation. There are lots of creams available on the market. You just have to get really good at reading labels and seeking professional advice. Some women experience an increase in vaginal or urinary infections. This can be exacerbated if you have other health issues such as diabetes.

You might find it hard to hold your urine long enough to get to the bathroom and you may find you are visiting the bathroom more frequently. You may also experience leakage during exercise, or when sneezing, coughing, laughing, running, or sexual intercourse.

And Speaking of Sex . . .

Around menopause, you may find that your feelings about sexual intercourse change quite drastically. When I was younger, I thought anyone over forty was dead from the neck down anyway and couldn't even imagine that they would still have feelings in this area or waste time thinking about it. I was wrong. You may find yourself less interested in sex, but I want to encourage you to make the effort since this could be some of the most satisfying times of intimacy you ever had. During this time, frequency may not be a feature, but quality can more than compensate for that.

At this stage in your relationship (if you have stayed open with each other), you have grown accustomed to one another and know the things you both like. This lays the groundwork for mutually-satisfying lovemaking that surpasses anything you experienced as newlyweds. To feel you are still attractive and knowing your partner desires you are mutually affirming, and orgasm and sexual release are invigorating.

Sex at this point does require time, effort, and planning. You shouldn't wait till last thing at night when you are both tired to engage in intercourse, since this can lead to frustrations and disappointment if you cannot rise to the occasion (no pun intended). Plan an afternoon get together with delight as your goal. Take your time and don't rush.

Make sure you have a light lunch with no garlic or onions unless you both have them and if you do, then prepare for the burp alert. Bring a supply of snacks to your room along with your choice of drinks, romantic candles (even though it may not be dark outside), and your favourite massage oils. You may want to book into a hotel but if not, make sure you have fresh sheets and the atmosphere in the bedroom is conducive for seduction. Kick everything off with a bubble bath and whatever is going to help you have a great experience. Please remember to lock your door if you have adult children who are still at home since they won't believe that it's possible for you to have sex in the afternoon and you may give them a heart attack if they walk in without knocking.

For some who due to ill health or disability may not be able to take part in penetrative sex, you can still give each other pleasure through kissing, fondling, stroking, and rubbing. Treat each other to a sensual massage using your favourite oils.

Touch is a powerful tool and as you each linger around those erogenous zones, you will give and experience pleasure. You need to learn what works for you and what your partner is open to. You and your spouse are still sexual beings and sexual partners and should seek to bring a level of satisfaction to each other. This will in turn affirm you as a person and allow you to feel a level of attractiveness and attraction to each other that will strengthen your marriage bond.

I know we took vows for better or for worse, but the worst should be that regardless of what you have both gone through, the default setting remains one of love and acceptance with a willingness to consider each other's needs for affection, acceptance, and expressed love. Find the will and energy from somewhere and I promise you it will pay dividends.

On the other side of the coin, it is possible for your libido to fall off the cliff edge as you experience a resurgence in your sex drive, with a corresponding return in levels of energy. This could be due to pregnancy no longer being a risk. You can stop worrying about becoming pregnant after one full year without a period. But remember, you can't ever stop protecting yourself against sexually-transmitted diseases (STDs), such as HIV/AIDS or gonorrhea. If you think you might be at risk of an STD, make sure your partner uses a condom each time you have intercourse.

Now that we have had our little talk about sex, it's time to get back to some of the other symptoms of this condition called menopause.

4)

SLEEP PROBLEMS

As mentioned earlier, you may start having trouble getting a good night's sleep while experiencing interruptions for one reason or another. Night sweats may awaken you and then have trouble falling back to sleep. Many a night I would wake up boiling hot, throw off the covers, and fall back to sleep, only to wake up an hour later freezing cold—and I mean tooth-chattering, shivering, plunged-in-ice-water cold. It would prove impossible to warm up and fall back to sleep, so I would be left longing for a hot flush to come along.

You may have retired feeling exhausted only to find you can't fall asleep easily, or you awaken too early. If this is because things are going around in your head and your brain can't seem to shut down, I suggest you do what I did. I would journal at night, make lists of all I needed to do the next day, even the smallest thing since it was so easy for me to forget. It's a good idea to avoid watching television or working on computers or iPads immediately before retiring since this activity impacts your ability to fall asleep. Reading a book can prove quite calming, as long as you are not reading an electronic book, which can have the same effect as watching television.

I usually have a time of winding down before I get into bed. This could just be puttering around in my bedroom preparing for the morning, checking my diary, listening to soothing music, taking a leisurely bath or shower, or having a warm nighttime drink. I purchased 100% cotton sheets (300 thread count) and made sure I established a nighttime routine.

If I still couldn't fall asleep, I would read a good book or listen to my favourite music, laying in the quiet and practicing what I call "soaking" in the peace. For a short span, play some non-directional music and position yourself in a comfortable position either lying down or in a comfy chair. As the music plays, imagine you are walking on a beach with Jesus during which time you get to ask Him one question and then listen for the answer.

Mood Changes

If you suffer from erratic sleep patterns around the time of menopause, you may find yourself becoming moody, irritable, or bad-tempered, or you may even suffer from acute depression. It's important to be aware of this possibility since you can be depressed and not even know it. Keep an eye on this so it does not develop into a chronic problem. It's not clear why this happens. I have not seen any research on whether there is a connection between changes in oestrogen levels and one's emotions.

Stress can be one of the causes, or family changes like grown children leaving the nest. You may feel redundant if you have centred your life around your children or neglected your relationship with your partner. Or you may have aging parents whilst at the same time holding down a demanding job. You may find yourself always feeling tired, and this could contribute to these mood changes. You may also feel emotionally fragile, crying when small children or animals appear on the TV.

If you have been experiencing extreme flushes or sweats, you may begin to isolate yourself because the feelings you experience seem to affect all your senses and may drain away your confidence. I described earlier how I began sweating profusely when I was speaking. I could feel the water running in my cleavage, down my arms, and onto my thighs. It was a major miracle that I didn't have a panic attack right there and then. I decided I would not speak or take engagements for several months. The reality was that speaking was not the problem; my changes were the problem. I realised that if I didn't take the bull by the horns, I might never go back to speaking.

Changes in Your Body

Your body is changing. Your waist tends to get larger as you lose muscle and gain fat. Your skin can get thinner. You might develop memory problems, and your joints and muscles may feel stiff and achy. This could be a result of having less oestrogen and growing older, so It's hard to differentiate between the two—getting older and menopause.

You may become more aware of smells around you

and on you as your sense of smell becomes more acute. You may start to smell things you never noticed before. You may start to dislike certain odours as they become stronger to you. Many women say they can no longer use certain products, including certain body care products they have used for years. Reactions range from feeling nauseous to being completely repulsed by the smells.

You may become more aware of your own body smells, and this can be quite disconcerting. Many women feel that their body odour is strong, so they resort to taking more frequent showers. Because they experience a raised awareness of their body, they feel everyone else is thinking they smell, too.

The PH in your vagina and some of your body fluids can start to emit a different odour, with the main change often in the vaginal area. Oestrogen actually causes the cervix to produce mucus in the vagina, and as your oestrogen levels fall during menopause, the production of mucus changes, which can either cause dryness, or for some women can actually increase the lubrication, and they worry because of the differences they feel.

Changes in vaginal mucus can also alter the balance of friendly bacteria in the vagina, and that can also affect the odour. With the vaginal fluids, you may find the amount changes, the colour changes, the smell changes, or the consistency changes as well. If you experience changes in vaginal mucus, especially if there's an odour or there's a distinct change in color, you will want to have this checked out by your GP.

The other main area where we sweat is under the arms, which often causes a lot of discomfort and distress because we can be sitting quite happily doing our jobs, and then think, "Oh, I can smell myself and my sweat." Remember, during menopause, especially if you're getting hot flashes or night sweats, you're going to sweat more anyway, which has other implications. The drop in oestrogen levels can affect the balance of bacteria on our skin, which can have an effect on the smells coming from under our arms.

Menopause can also stress the liver. It also slows down the digestive system and metabolic rate, so our bowels can become a bit sluggish and we end up with constipation. When this happens, the body has to find other ways of getting rid of toxins, and one of the places happens to be under the arms. Even if you're using antiperspirants or deodorants, you can start to smell a bit more earlier in the day than usual.

If you are getting a bit smelly under the arms, or if you are experiencing bloating, digestive discomforts, or constipation, remember that constipation can also give you bad breath. By supporting your liver through drinking lots of water (with a slice of lemon), you can help with detoxification, ease bowel movements, and help restore regular bowel motions. Also, do not start showering yourself three or four times a day because that will seriously disrupt the balance of friendly bacteria under the arms. Simply try using a slightly stronger deodorant.

Changes to Your Heart and Bones

I don't want to alarm or overwhelm you, but at the same time you are experiencing the above-mentioned changes, there are changes to your heart and bones. Some of these may happen without you even noticing.

Osteoporosis

Every day you are alive, your body is busy breaking down old bone and replacing it with new healthy bone. Oestrogen helps to control bone loss. Since we lose oestrogen around the time of menopause, we also lose bone faster than we can replace it. Over time, we lose bone density and our bones become weaker and may break more easily. This is the condition known as osteoporosis. A visit to your doctor can help address this change. The doctor may suggest you have a bone density test to find out if you are developing this problem. Your doctor can also suggest ways to prevent or treat osteoporosis.

Heart Disease

After menopause, women are more likely to succumb to heart disease, and changes in their levels of oestrogen can be part of the cause. Of course, simply getting older can cause this as well. As we age, we may develop other problems, such as high blood pressure or obesity, which puts us at greater risk of heart disease. Gaining weight doesn't help with bone density problems either and adds increased pressure to our knee and hip joints.

The added weight can hurt our ego, too. I remember being weighed at the doctor's office and he promptly informed me that I was grossly obese. I quickly informed him that I was grossly insulted. He was unaware of the fact that I had very large bones! Please be meticulous about having your health checkups and watch your blood pressure, cholesterol levels, and blood sugars, and don't neglect your breast screening or cervical smear.

There is a good reason why menopause is referred to as "change of life," because there are so many changes that take place. Let's continue to look at those changes in the next chapter.

Other Changes to Look For

If you have not paid attention to yourself in your life, it is imperative that you look after yourself and have good self-care during this season of change. If you have left a proper regime of caring for yourself until now, it's not too late to start. Hopefully your children are grown so some of the time you used to lavish on them can now be spent on you.

I have found just the act of getting older can lead to loss of confidence, competence, and self-esteem unless you take steps to avoid them. I have also found that this is the right time to take life by the horns and be intentional about what you would like to happen. Perhaps for the first time in a long time, you get to determine who and what you will be. Your options may be limited but you still have quite a few.

Allowing extra time for the things you need to do will help reduce your stress levels. Stress is your number one enemy and affects every system in your body with the reduction of oestrogen and progesterone, you will feel the impact of stress far more than before. Build in time for your monthly massages, as well as time for prayer and meditation. Here are some other changes you may experience and these may surprise and even startle you if they occur.

Changes to Your Skin

During and more so towards the end of peri-menopause, you may experience extreme itching caused by dryness of the skin over your entire body, especially your scalp, neck/chest area, thighs, and upper arms. The skin over your entire body becomes dry and soaks up moisturiser. You may have to reapply moisturiser several times during the day. It is better to use a cream rather than a lotion since the latter tend to be watery. Use a moisturising body wash as opposed to soap, which can be really drying.

Changes to Your Hair

As you go through this stage, you will notice that your hair changes and may become thinner and brittle, breaking easily. Your scalp can become itchy and sensitive to heat. What used to be routine blow drying becomes torture as the heat hits your scalp. Sitting under the dryer isn't much better as again the heat is intense. I had to start using treatment to add moisture to my hair.

Changes to Your Nails

My nails became extremely sensitive and would break or peel off after flaking. I had to stop using things like acrylic and shellac nail polishes as they seemed to exacerbate the problems I was having with dryness.

Changes to Your Teeth

During this period of time, your teeth can become more sensitive and may weaken. I broke three teeth in a period of a few months, and I wasn't even chewing anything hard. Your gums may also start receding or become more sensitive, bleeding when you brush. Thinning of your bones does not just take place in your long bones but can also happen in your jaw bones, so this may affect your teeth and cause them to loosen in the jaw. This together with receding gums can hasten tooth loss. Watch out for bad breath, too.

Keeping your routine every six-month dental appointment now becomes more important than ever. Brushing well, using the right kind of toothpaste, and maybe switching to an electric toothbrush might be helpful. I found it much easier to clean my back teeth and achieved a much cleaner feel with the electric brush.

Threading Waxing for Hair Removal

To get rid of excessive hair, especially

on my neck and chin, threading and waxing proved to be the best method and left my skin feeling soft and blemish free. This would last about two weeks before it would need to be done again. Threading and waxing were much better than shaving since shaving tends to cause hairs either to be ingrown or to grow back thicker and darker.

Weight and Diet

It is harder to lose weight during and after menopause, so it makes sense to develop a healthy diet and eating habits. Eating more protein and reducing carbohydrates and sugars (including fruit sugars) will help. Eat more green leafy vegetables, too.

Exercise

You don't necessarily have to join a gym or do exercises you don't enjoy. Simply walking for up to 30 or 40 minutes, three or four times a week, would be sufficient to increase your heart rate and build your muscle density. This is the ability to reproduce a particular movement without conscious thought, acquired as a result of frequent repetition of that movement.

Set regular times for your exercise and make it a part of your routine. Exercise will strengthen your muscles, as well as increase your stamina and metabolic rate. This means that even when you are resting, you are burning more calories than if you had not exercised.

I mentioned above that your lifestyle may have caused you to pay attention to your family's needs and not your own. This could easily have become a habit without you realizing it. Therefore, it is important that during your change you become proactive where you are concerned. This may be the greatest and most difficult change you encounter, but it is important. In the next chapter, I will discuss the importance of having a good support team of relationships around you to help you through this difficult time, and of setting new life goals to ensure your own mental health and well-being.

6

Relationships & Well-Being

Please ensure that you make setting fresh goals an integral part of your life. For me it became a priority to have things laid out in an orderly manner. As I examined my life, I realised I did not want to be weighed down with things like belongings, clothes, or gadgets. This was the right time for me to simplify my life and relationships.

I learned how much my family and friends I had really mattered to me, and I also concluded that other people needed to earn a place in my life. I didn't have time to waste with individuals who only wanted to take advantage of or abuse my friendship. It was during this season that I became a grandmother for the first time.

My eldest child had been pregnant several times but lost her first child quite early on and also lost twin boys at around twenty weeks. She then lost a girl named Jada at around the twenty-one-week mark.

Jada was the first time I had been able to hold one of my grandchildren, even though she lived for only six hours. It was too early for us to do anything to save her. I remember holding her with tears in my eyes trying to cram a lifetime of love into her, as I watched her move her tiny arms and legs, knowing it was only a matter of time before she would leave us. I am not able to convert my feelings of devastation into words, both for myself and my husband. And we had such pain for our daughter and her husband, who were experiencing extreme trauma, having lost four babies and wondering if they would ever be parents.

During this time, we stayed in our support orbit, trying not to make it about us but to keep hope in their hearts and reassuring them that they would be parents one day. Rather than all this driving us apart as a family, each experience cemented us together. As we stood over the tiny white coffins of each burial, we had feelings we never knew we would experience, much less survive. Our faith in God's goodness was our anchor, our life jacket, and coast guard.

When my daughter told us she was pregnant again, we held our breath for nine months, praying one long prayer the entire time. We held on to our trust in God with all we had, for another loss would not just be the loss of a grandchild but the loss of a daughter. You cannot imagine how we felt when Jade Zara Lee came into the world on October 7, 2016, the same date as her grandfather's birthday.

Good Mental Health

Because of the work I do, I get to witness the internal workings of many marriages. Women who have pushed on through their marriages despite struggles and shortfalls in the balance of the relationship actually find themselves questioning a lot of things about their lives as they navigated this period in their lives. It is as though menopause is a crossroads of sorts.

Many women have coped with rejection, put-downs, and sometimes outright cruelty in their marriages and relationships. For many reasons, they put up with the situation, sometimes due to concern about their children being from a broken home, fear of being a single parent, or for fear of appearing to be a failure. Any woman in this stage of life is looking for acceptance, genuine affection, and affirmation in her marriage.

During menopause, there can be issues with confidence and self-esteem. A wife needs her attractiveness affirmed. She needs to know she is loved, desired, and still has an active role to play in her husband's life. After having had a few children, maybe her figure has taken a hit. She held down a job at the same time as raising a family, running a home, and trying to keep it all together.

One of the things that was right in my face during this time was the fact I was not getting younger but getting older and did not have as many years before me a I had behind me. This really served to focus and clarify my thinking, increasing the need to have active goals and make a concerted effort to leave a legacy.

It is during this time that many women learn to support and love themselves. It's wonderful to have someone who loves and supports you, but what do you do if you do not have that significant other? You learn to love yourself, care for yourself, and optimise your health. I recommend a full-body massage at least once a month. This will help relieve stress, release toxins from your system, and cause you to relax at a new level.

Set goals for your water intake, exercise, weight loss, and rest. Any new habit needs control and maintenance if it is going to be sustained. Any new habit that we want to be part of our lives going forward has to be built into our routine. Set goals for your grooming care along with a monthly budget for it. Pay attention to your skin care, make up, grooming, and the coordination of your clothing. Dress comfortably but appropriately for any appointment, event, or occasion you are attending in your home or outside.

Work and the Menopause

The type of work you do can also be directly affected during this time. You have to continue to maintain the high levels of excellence you're used to, even when you're experiencing hot flushes, irritability, and the numerous other symptoms I described above. If your job involves giving public presentations, you may find you become more anxious than usual. Many women resign from their jobs because of this type of pressure. It's rare that male colleagues or husbands actually understand what women are experiencing, and many women feel unsupported during this time.

Unfortunately, we tend to blame ourselves rather than realising there is something intrinsically wrong with the system in which we are forced to live and work. No man experiencing the symptoms of menopause would actually expect to keep pushing forward and working as normal. Some women leave their jobs or even go part time and take a position with less prestige just to be able to maintain a work life. This is a good time for us to look at our work-life balance.

It Will End

After many years going through the symptoms I've talked about, it was such a surprise one day to wake up and actually feel my energy return and that life was really worth living. I felt I had some control again. This mid-life event is a time of reflection and I found myself wanting to add value, not just to myself but also to those around me. I accepted that I was older, but it was still possible for me to step onto the world stage and fulfil the calling on my life.

This period is the time when you can have a more effective focus, for you have some experience under your belt, have some things to say, and can devote the time to make it happen that otherwise went to family. Of course, the backdrop always has to be one of self-care with times of preparation, learning to pace yourself to get everything done you now have on your list of goals.

That wraps us my experience and research on peri-menopause and menopause. Next, I want to include some of the stories I have collected from my friends who share their own perspective, experience, and tips for survival during the change of life.

ENHANCERS – STORIES FROM OTHER LADIES

1. My Story

I was around the age of 50 when I began to feel changes in my body. At the same time, I was diagnosed with hyperthyroidism (an overactive thyroid), which increases the effects of menopausal symptoms.

First, my period became light and irregular, and then the hot flushes came. It started as if a bucket of heat was poured over me, which ran halfway down my body for what seemed to last a few minutes. This would happen gradually but frequently during the day—every day. The night sweats came with a vengeance, with sweat rolling off my nose, causing me to change the sheets every night. Insomnia became the norm, and so I became forgetful at times due to fatigue. I would lose my ability to concentrate and I thought people saw me as strange or drunk because I found myself not putting my sentences together properly.

My husband had no interest in learning about menopause at all because he was not going through this experience himself. He could not understand why I would resist him when it came to our sexual relationship. I had vaginal dryness, so intercourse became painful. Therefore, our sexual relationship eventually had to end because it was impossible to go through the pain and I was not able to commit to his demands any longer.

Even though I was going through this season, I regularly said to myself that I would not take hormone replacement therapy (HRT) because it would not stop the menopause, it would only suppress it. After all, God created men and woman in His own image and it was good (see Genesis

1:27) and we are fearfully and wonderfully made (see Psalms 139:14). Therefore, I believe that we should go through the process without defiling our bodies with medicines that will mess up our hormones. I concluded there must be a reason why God made us this way, so I decided to ride out the storm, going through the highs and the lows of moods, which lasted almost ten years. Now the storm is over and to be honest, I never really noticed when it had calmed down. After ten years, one day I suddenly realised, "Oh, I feel better."

I have learnt that menopause can increase the risk of developing osteoporosis (weak bones) as a result of the lower level of oestrogen in the body, of which I have recently been diagnosed. Eating a healthy diet, including plenty of fruit, vegetables, and regular exercise and keeping active are advised. Consume sources of calcium, such as low-fat milk and yoghurt. Vitamin D helps to keep the bones strong. This helps to alleviate menopausal symptoms. — *Elizabeth Johnson (married with four children, living in the West Midlands, United Kingdom)*

2. Wow, the Menopause!

As I was growing up, I was not aware of what my mother went through as she moved from her forties into her fifties. How I wish that had been different, for I would be a lot better equipped to handle this stage of my life. Yet in saying that, I think I have had the best example of someone who had only just started menopause a couple of years before I met her, and this person was Pastor Yvonne Brooks. I watched her in amazement as she got up to speak, preach, or teach, and as passionate as she was in her delivery, so was she passionate in the way she embraced her hot flushes.

I would watch as perspiration would start at her brow and then trickle down her face. At times she would stop in mid-sentence and lose her train of thought. She always made that '1.5 minutes' (I know how long it took because I learnt to time mine) either theatrical or humorous, or used it as a teaching point. In all three instances, I learned to appreciate the next stage of womanhood and wondered how long it would be before I got there.

I noticed the meetings I attended had women often bringing out fans, some made out of material elaborate and beautifully decorated, others practical ones that were wooden or plastic. I observed hand-held, battery-operated fans coming out of handbags, women asking for a window to be opened or a fan switched on, and I marveled that the body could heat up and explode in such a short space of time. I watched as layers of clothes would come off and then they would go back on and I was intrigued. About three months ago, I noticed that I would be sitting on the sofa and all of a sudden, I would feel a warm glow move over my body.

At first, it was comfortable and I would just express that it was a tad warm in the house. As time progressed, I noticed that this feeling would come and go with a little more intensity than the last time. One day at work, I decided to see if I indeed had 'entered' *the* menopause stage and when I began to feel warm, I timed the feeling until it ended, and it lasted 1.5 minutes.

I must admit it was an amazing experience and I was so in awe of it that I wanted it to come back (I must say I tried hard to concentrate and focus internally, hoping I could 'magically' cause it to re-occur). It started off like I had a fleece on and went into a heated room. It was just a small change and then it began to move, from my waistline all the way up my body, down through my arms, and then up my neck and through my head, where it disappeared like steam (I imagined opening the valve on a pressure cooker and letting out the steam).

Throughout the 12 weeks (until now), I have monitored its progress, and I must share that one cold winter's day, I left work huddled up in my scarf and coat pulled tightly around me. The wind was howling and it was quite chilly. As I walked,

I began to feel the rise of that familiar heat and I started smiling because I embraced it as a godsend—my own internal heater. What I didn't anticipate was the increase in temperature. I'm not sure if all the layers of clothes added to the heat, but all of a sudden, it felt like I was a pot on a gas stove and the flame was increased to high.

In that moment, I did something I wouldn't normally do and that was pull off the scarf, unbutton my coat, and walk directly into the icy cold wind. To be honest, I felt like a superhero! With the icy wind attacking me and my inferno blasting out, my imagination played out to the fullest as I opened my arms wide like MJ did in his video, *Earth Song*, and walked in the middle of the High Street embracing the cold air. As quickly as it had built up, it disappeared, and I once again found myself putting on my scarf and pulling my coat tighter around me, bending my head to cut through the icy blast. It was an exhilarating experience.

Sometimes I just sit and when I feel

the familiar rise of heat starting, I try to beat it by removing my cardigan or gown as quickly as I can. I then just sit calmly and let it wash over me. To be honest, I find it quite therapeutic. I say, *I'm not having a hot flush. It's more like I'm having a short, private holiday in tropical-like conditions.* It doesn't quite work that way, however, when I'm in meetings serving as the note taker. I find myself having to make important decisions, like try to concentrate on what the speaker is saying whilst feeling as though I'm going to explode and set the room alight, or take the agenda and fold into a paper fan and furiously try to put out the rising fire under my skin, totally missing vital information for the meeting.

This week I'm experiencing a new sensation. As my temperatures rise, I'm watching the creases in my hands turn red and I'm noticing that not only is the heat intense but I'm beginning to perspire with little beads of water forming on my forehead, the nape of my neck, under my breasts and behind my knees (the sensation has also descended from my waist to my thighs and knees). The duration of each hot flush remains the same, but they are becoming more frequent.

So far, I've had my first experience during the winter months, My journey will take me into summer and I'm wondering how that will play out, the heat from within and without. I'm definitely going to be *hot stuff* or I could literally sing like Alesha Keys, "This girl is on fire," and not be joking.

On a more serious note, has the menopause affected me emotionally, physically, mentally? It has contributed to the other changes I am going through in conjunction with an upcoming birthday on which I'll be turning 50. I'm becoming more reflective and I'm really starting to enjoy my own company more. I'm comfortable with who I am. I've become a lot more health-and-body conscious, so I have changed my diet and started exercising.

I've realised that I can still have fun and be spiritual. My relationship with the

Father has deepened and the Scriptures have become more important to me. My spiritual journey has taken me to places I was scared to go——to look within and to love and embrace even the negatives and the shadows. I've decided that I don't need the mask anymore, and I don't need to consistently ask or seek permission to do something I want to do.

I've stopped going on guilt trips and have jumped off the fast train of life to rather catch the bus and enjoy the scenery. Sometimes I'm hesitant and sometimes I feel confused and sometimes I feel tearful, while at other times, I'm so happy and filled with such intense joy that I feel I'm going to explode into twins. I'm singing more, dancing more, and laughing more, but above all, I'm grateful for every stage of my life.

I've looked at menopause from a medical point of view and I understand what is happening to my body and have relayed any concerns to my GP. I'm guessing that as I travel further into my journey,

I'll have to perhaps start taking supplements, drinking more herbal teas, and relying on the experiences of others who have travelled this journey before me. Overall, I encourage anyone who is about to start this journey to journal, share your experience, and speak to someone who is going through or has gone through it, since it will be different for everyone. I have found that the menopause is a subject that's not really spoken about. We just seem to quietly reach for the fan in our bags and furiously try to create a mini-tornado to cool us down. — *Anonymous, divorced with one child.*

3. My Menopause

Looking back, my menopausal symptoms began when I was around 45 or 46 years old, but it took a while for me to recognise what was going on. I began having night sweats that prompted me to go to see my GP. As I was still having regular menstrual periods, he sent me to see the nurse to have bloods taken. The initial thought was that I had a thyroid disorder, but the result came back as borderline, so my GP told me to monitor how things went. Managing a family along with a busy and demanding job, the night sweats came and went, and I got on with life.

Fast forward a couple of years when my periods gradually became irregular, sometimes light and other times heavy. The longest lasted six weeks, which prompted my GP to prescribe progesterone tablets for me. I was only able to take one tablet because they made me feel really nauseous—just like early pregnancy sickness. Further blood tests taken showed the levels of oestrodiol in my blood indicated that I was peri-menopausal. I had my very last menstrual period at age 48.

I was sad when my periods stopped. It wasn't something I ever thought I would miss but I did. It marked an end to something that would not return. I took my fertility for granted. I was never going to have any more children, but at that point, the choice was gone. I was now a woman of a certain age, less desirable, less visible, less relevant. Well, that's how it felt at the time.

Menopausal Symptoms

I cannot remember exactly when the hot flushes began, but they had become a regular and distressing feature of my life for years. The heat seemed to come up from my feet, and by the time it reached my head area, I would feel uncomfortable, hot, and what can only be described as panicky. They would last a few seconds or a few minutes, once a day or several times a day, and they always took me by surprise. The flushes at night would wake me up, and when they did, the duvet got kicked off and any nightclothes taken off as quickly as possible. At their worst, I kept a cold, wet flannel on the headboard to mop up the sweat and cool my skin, along with a glass of iced water nearby.

On more than one occasion, I leapt out of bed and hung out of the open window in order to cool down——in the middle of the night with no clothes on. At moments like that, getting cool was the number one priority. Waking up sometime later shivering with cold, I had to retrieve the discarded duvet from the floor, which happened often. Later, I invested in a remote-controlled tower fan that I could put on a timer and operate from my bed if needed. Twelve years on, the fan is still in my bedroom and is still used occasionally.

The unpredictability of the hot flushes was at worst distressing, at best inconvenient. Just looking at a roll neck jumper could sometimes trigger a hot flush or power surge as I sometimes called them. I soon learned that wearing layers was the answer. Being able to remove jumpers and other top layers of clothing quickly while remaining decent in public was important.

Other symptoms included forgetfulness, which surprised and frightened me. I forgot colleague's names, including people I had worked with for years. I remember having to ask a colleague what another colleague's name was since I was too embarrassed to ask them myself. Around this time, my own mother had been diagnosed and was suffering from Alzheimer's disease and my personal life was in turmoil; I couldn't figure out if I was just exhausted with life or if I also had dementia. I didn't go to the GP because I was afraid of what he might say. I often felt like there was a black cloud over my head wherever I went. Feeling emotional and in a bad mood for no good reason was also a common occurrence. Around this time, I also started gaining weight I had trouble getting rid of.

Things that Worked for Me

There came a time when I felt that I had to regain control of my body. I read a lot about the subject. I spoke to female friends about their experiences of the menopause. Working in a female-dominated workplace provided me with plenty of anecdotal remedies, supplements to take, therapies to try, foods and drinks to consume and avoid, HRT or not, patches or tablets.

I decided early on that HRT would

be a last option for me. I didn't want to medicate a natural phase of my life. I had medicated my fertility, but it just didn't feel right for me to do the same for the menopause. I had many friends who were taking HRT in one form or another who found it invaluable, so I knew that if I needed it, it was an option. I thought about my mother and her peers. It wouldn't have crossed her mind to go to see her doctor about her hot flushes. She managed to get through it and so would I.

I tried several things—supplements such as wild yam, black cohosh, and raspberry leaf tea, but sage tablets were the most effective. The hot flushes stopped almost immediately after I started to take them and provided a blessed relief, but like most things I tried, the relief was temporary. By the second packet, the hot flushes returned. Next up was eating tofu: tofu curry, stew, stir fry, etc. Every meal, I made with tofu in it provided a relief from the hot flushes that night, but I just couldn't eat tofu every day.

Acupuncture was a surprise discovery. It was painless and effective at reducing the hot flushes almost immediately, along with drinking the Chinese tea that came with it. My periods even restarted months after they had stopped, but I couldn't keep up with the acupuncture even though it worked because I couldn't afford it. I would have liked to have tried reflexology sessions but at the time I couldn't have afforded keeping up with those sessions either.

Drinking ice cold sparkling water always helped. There were never enough ice cubes in the freezer so I bought bags of them from the freezer section in the supermarket so I never ran out. Whenever I went out, I'd be prepared: layered clothing, bottle of cold water, and being prepared to say, "Can I open the window please?!"

Twelve Years On

I still have occasional hot flushes, but they are nowhere near as intense as they once were. It took far too long for me to recognise that coffee, red wine, weight gain, and too much sugar are triggers for a hot flush even now. Knowing this back then could have made life a little less uncomfortable.

The brain fog/forgetfulness/black cloud eventually lifted. It is difficult to know when that happened or if anything I did or didn't do contributed to that. I was just grateful that it wasn't permanent. I was also pleased that I didn't need to take HRT for my symptoms. What concerned me about HRT was how long would I have to take it and would the hot flushes return with a vengeance? There was no way of knowing.

Being informed about the menopause was important. I needed to understand what was happening and why. Speaking to other women who had experienced it or who were going through it at the same time as I was a massive help and support. – *W. Carroll, May 2019 (divorced with two children living in Stafford, United Kingdom)*

4. Another Account

My life changed forever when my baby girl was born. I was 42 years young and slowly moving toward menopause. My sisters and I always talked about how our mother made getting older appear to be an effortless experience. It was quite the contrary for me! I remember the mood swings, weight gain, and all the physical discomforts. My explanation for suddenly sweating like a pig on a hot tin roof was, "Excuse me, I'm having a personal summer." Prayerfully, I made it through. I remember the crying spells over the most trivial reasons. This reminded me of my Thespian days in high school. Not to be defeated by these radical changes, I used those tears to intercede. My life lesson learned could be summarized by the words of a proverbial author who said, "Life is like a bowl of cherries, but remember the pits."

I was able to survive all of the menopausal discomfort by taking it one day at a time. I remember reading and researching as much information as I could about this change taking place in my body. Knowledge was powerful for me. Prayers became more intense and sharing my experiences with my sisters made it more bearable. My baby even helped to distract and focus my attention on caring for her. My biggest disappointment was the weight gain. With prayer, however, I made the adjustments. I refused to take the HRT due to the possible side effects. Nevertheless, I made it through. Laughter was my best friend along with being totally honest with myself and my hubby. His understanding of my transition helped tremendously. — *Mrs. Lynda Hughes (wife and mother living in the U.S.A.)*

5. My Menopause Experience

My experience of menopause was a dramatic one. It was unexpected and I was younger than most when it happened. This meant that my dream of having a second child was shattered. I became unwell and overwhelmed with the symptoms of menopause such as hot flushes, aches, fatigue, heavy night sweats, and a weakened bladder. Along the way, I found it difficult to retain my urine. I could visit the toilets between five and ten times within an hour. I saw my GP as a matter of urgency, and she prescribed some tablets that helped alleviate most of the symptoms. Furthermore, I embarked on a personal research binge. I began to read about healthy diet and how I could incorporate this into my eating habits. I stopped eating food that would trigger hot flushes and other symptoms.

I resolved to change my diet and began to eat specific types of vegetables, fruits, and juices. (Please see separate list below.) I also made it a custom to take some multivitamins, coupled with prayer of course. I began to notice significant positive changes in my body. I felt much better and healthier. I also noticed a meaningful reduction of the episodes of hot flushes. Similarly, I started to do physical exercise and this helped alleviate the fatigue, aches, and hot flushes. In addition, I did some Kegel exercise twice a day, which helped strengthen my bladder.

With prayer, I have reached a place where I had to accept this change knowing "that all things work together for good for those who love the Lord and are called according to His purpose" (Romans 8:28). Although, my dream of having a second child might have been shattered, God is still good no matter what and I have learned to appreciate Him for the one child He has given me when I remember that there is someone out there who would do anything to have even one. I have learned to count my blessings. The following is not meant to be an exhaustive list.

Hot flash trigger food

- Alcohol
- Chocolate
- Caffeinated drinks
- Dairy products
- Spicy dishes
- Fried food

- Excess sugar
- Meat products

Foods that relieve hot flashes

- Oily Fish (sardines)
- Eggs
- Leafy green vegetables (kale, spinach, watercress, broccoli, cabbage, cauliflower etc.)
- Flaxseeds
- Whole-grain food (brown rice, oatmeal, barley, etc.
- Chickpeas
- A glass of pure or organic pomegranate juice once a day.

I encourage you to watch your diet, for what you eat can alleviate or aggravate your physical symptoms. — *Anonymous (divorced with one daughter)*

6. An Unusual Symptom

I don't even know when I started the menopause because it took me a while before I realized *this thing* was happening to me. When I was out shopping with my sister one day, I got so hot and in a state of physical discomfort that I wanted to rip my clothes off. I couldn't get the first layer off quickly enough. As if it made any difference, my skin was still piping hot, but with no flames to be seen. My sister kept me distracted with her laughing and pleading with me not to take off any more clothes. "Girl, you have it bad," she said.

It was then I realised I was going through the menopause for real. This carried on for as long as I can remember, with various other symptoms that I learned can all be connected to the menopause. I experienced night sweats, lack of energy, tender and bloating stomach, elevated heart rate, tender breasts, irregular periods, and loss of memory. I couldn't remember anything, so a pen and a diary became an integral part of my life. I said to people, "If it's not in my diary, it ain't happening," and, believe me, that's not a joke or a myth. It's a fact.

One of the most worrying thing for me was at around 50 years old, I was in a consultation with my GP who expressed her surprise that I was still having a full period term. Of course, I was shocked that she was shocked, and I began to wonder if something was wrong with me.

Not long after my cycle stopped for almost a year. *Praise the Lord and thank You, Jesus*, I thought. But after about a year, there it was again the "Lady from red hills" (my period) had returned—every month, some two or three days at a time. The GP told me it wasn't uncommon for this to happen, so I lived with it and it has done so ever since. Sometimes there is nothing showing for months except the usual physical and mental symptoms described earlier.

I have had other symptoms, but I am not sure how they might be connected, things like impaired vision, diminished hearing loss, weakened bones, hair loss, soft nails that breaks easily, feelings of depression, anxiety and, yes let's go there, loss of interest in sex. In all of this, my husband has been lovingly supportive.

The years go by and at every turn I have been looking for support from other women my age and those who are older. I have so many questions: *What is it like for you? What was your experience? How did you cope? Did you finish early or did you continue as late as I have? Was there or is there a remedy?*

I haven't finished yet so even at 65 and still like clockwork, I have a seven-, sometimes a nine-day period, which leaves me feeling like there is something wrong. I sometimes remind people (and myself) that I look young for my age, so my body thinks it's young and is behaving like it's young. Whatever the reason, I still have a menstrual cycle at my age, and I don't know why or when they will finish.

The GPs have no answers for me. They have checked and tested and carried out two separate operations within the last seven years. They say I have unusually thick walls but there is no sign of cancer. (Thank You, Jesus.) The doctors can (as a way of solving but not curing the problem) insert a marina coil to block the menstruation. I have not accepted this offer to date since I don't believe blocking is the thing to do.

So you see ladies, sharing your story and me sharing mine can only help us better manage these delicate years of our lives. The lack of information/support and open conversation left me in the dark to struggle with something I didn't understand. It was like my own body covered me with a warm blanket and I felt safe and protected, but then something subtly dragged the blanket off me, leaving me exposed and at the mercy of these psychological symptoms I did not understand.

It has been a very long process to date, and for me, there is no end in sight. Writing about my story, however, has helped put things into perspective, I hope sharing my story will help other women come to terms with what we classify under the umbrella "The Change." — *T.M.S., married with three adult children, Birmingham*

Appendix

Q: What exact changes are taking place hormonally in the menopause?

Your levels of oestrogen are dropping. Progesterone and testosterone also decrease but they don't have the same impact as low levels of oestrogen.

For more details see:

https://www.google.co.uk/amp/s/www.bbc.co.uk/news/amp/health48258910

Read the following sections:

- So what's behind the change?
- Are other hormones involved?

Q: What does oestrogen do?

Oestrogen is crucial to the whole monthly reproductive cycle: the development and release of an egg from the ovaries each month for fertilisation and the thickening of the lining of the womb ready to accept the fertilised egg.

Oestrogen

- supports bone health and strength
- Helps to regulate our bodies temperature as it is involved in how our body manages changes in temperature
- The hormone interacts with chemicals in brain receptors which control mood, and at low levels it can cause anxiety and low mood.

Source:

https://www.google.co.uk/amp/s/www.bbc.co.uk/news/amp/health48258910

Read the following section:

- What impact do hormonal changes have?

Q: What does progesterone do?

Progesterone helps to prepare the

body for pregnancy every month, and it declines when periods stop.

Source:

https://www.google.co.uk/amp/s/www.bbc.co.uk/news/amp/health48258910

Q: Are there natural or herbal treatments for hot flushes?

1. Soy: There is quite a bit of evidence that soy products can alleviate hot flashes, but the degree of relief provided varies widely. In general, soy high in diadzein is most effective. Diadzein is a compound that can be converted in the intestines to equol, a chemical that attaches to estrogen receptors to duplicate some of estrogen's effects in the body. However, because only about 50% of Asian and 25% Caucasian women carry the intestinal bacteria necessary to produce equol from daidzein,

equol supplements may be more effective than soy. There is early evidence that a 10-milligram S-equol supplement taken twice a day may control hot flashes with no harmful side effects. However, more studies are needed to better determine its effectiveness.'

2. Herbal remedies: Although several nonhormonal treatments for menopause are often recommended, there is not enough evidence from clinical studies to recommend them. These include lifestyle changes like getting more exercise or practicing yoga, deep breathing, or relaxation techniques. *Nor, despite scores of studies, is there convincing evidence that widely used herbal remedies like black cohosh, dong quai, ginseng, and wild yam are effective,* either (emphasis added).

Source:

https://www.health.
harvard.edu/menopause/
nonhormonal-treatments-for-menopause

a. Black Cohosh: This North American traditional herb can help hot flushes although never as well as HRT. Black cohosh does not help with anxiety or low mood, but black cohosh can interact with other medicines and there are unknown risks regarding safety'

b. St. John's Wort: Again, the good news is that St John's Wort was shown to have benefit in relieving vasomotor symptoms, particularly in women with a history of, or at high risk of breast cancer. However, like black cohosh, it does interact with other drugs which again makes it a drug we have concerns about, including its reliability regarding dose effectiveness and safety profiles. Women on tamoxifen must not take St John's Wort as it makes the tamoxifen ineffective.

c. Other herbal treatments including Ginseng and Chinese herbal medicines are not shown to improve hot flushes, anxiety or low mood.'

3. Acupuncture: Studies showed no difference in women who received acupuncture compared with those who received sham acupuncture, but there is a very high placebo effect with both sham and real acupuncture.

Source:

https://www.womens-health-concern.
org/help-and-advice/factsheets/
complementaryalternative-therapies-
menopausal-women

4. Diet: Maintaining and heathy diet and exercise appear to be the best natural way to stay healthy through the menopause.

Source:

https://www.nutrition.org.uk/healthyliving/lifestages/menopause

5. Other sources of information on the menopause:

https://my.clevelandclinic.org/health/diseases/15224-menopause-perimenopause-and-postmenopause

https://m.acog.org/Patients/FAQs/The-Menopause-Years?IsMobileSet=true

https://www.nhs.uk/conditions/menopause/

https://www.bupa.co.uk/health-information/womens-health/menopause

Pastor Yvonne E. Brooks

Yvonne Elizabeth Brooks is the first assistant pastor of New Jerusalem Apostolic Church——a thriving church that is having a huge impact in the community in the city of Birmingham. She is a qualified Behavioural Consultant, Mental Health Nurse and Registered General Nurse and from this, she has a passion for seeing people receive deliverance, healing, and restoration.

Pastor Yvonne has completed a Bachelor's Degree in Biblical Studies and a Doctorate in Theology and Biblical Studies as testament to her desire to grow and develop so she can be a blessing to others as she delivers the Word nationally and internationally. She has also presented on television and radio and is the author of two books: *Touching God's Heart: Prayers that Make a Difference* and *Purpose Steps.* As a result of her ongoing service, she has been recognised with a number of awards including the Women of Excellence Trailblazer Award.

Her main achievement is being the founder and director of Women of Purpose Ministries, which inspires women around the globe to become women of purpose so they can take their place on the world stage. WOP is a ministry that encompasses a number of life-changing programmes, including the Women of Purpose Conference, Esther's International Program, Esther's Extra, NEXT Steps, EXCEL, Ambassador, and Tohorah (a retreat for teenagers). Her desire is to help others to transform life's broken places to a place of lifelong fulfilment and purpose. (To learn more, please visit her website at http://esthersacademy.co.uk).

The greatest achievement of her life

is her beautiful family, which has stemmed from over four decades of marriage to Bishop M.A. Brooks. Together they have three talented children and two grandchildren, Jade and Zion.

Made in the USA
Monee, IL
07 July 2026

56551599R00056